46 Meal Recipes to Solve Your Constipation Problems:

Improve Your Digestion through Intelligent Food Choices and Well Organized Meal Recipes

By

Joe Correa CSN

COPYRIGHT

This publication is designed to provide accurate and authoritative information in regard to the subject matter covered. It is sold with the understanding that neither the author nor the publisher is engaged in rendering medical advice. If medical advice or assistance is needed, consult with a doctor. This book is considered a guide and should not be used in any way detrimental to your health. Consult with a physician before starting this nutritional plan to make sure it's right for you.

ACKNOWLEDGEMENTS

This book is dedicated to my friends and family that have had mild or serious illnesses so that you may find a solution and make the necessary changes in your life.

46 Meal Recipes to Solve Your Constipation Problems:

Improve Your Digestion through Intelligent Food Choices and Well Organized Meal Recipes

By

Joe Correa CSN

CONTENTS

ABOUT THE AUTHOR

After years of Research, I honestly believe in the positive effects that proper nutrition can have over the body and mind. My knowledge and experience has helped me live healthier throughout the years and which I have shared with family and friends. The more you know about eating and drinking healthier, the sooner you will want to change your life and eating habits.

Nutrition is a key part in the process of being healthy and living longer so get started today. The first step is the most important and the most significant.

INTRODUCTION

46 Meal Recipes to Solve Your Constipation Problems: Improve Your Digestion through Intelligent Food Choices and Well Organized Meal Recipes

By Joe Correa CSN

Constipation is a very common problem throughout the world and everybody experiences it once in a while. Approximately 42 million people have problems with constipation. We all have different habits when going to the toilet. Still, for some people, once or twice a week is a totally normal thing but ideally you should be going to the bathroom atleast once a day.

The most common simptoms for constipation are stomach cramps, being unable to empty your bowels, or extremely hard stool. This can have psychological affects that are followed by loss of appetite and anxiety.

Irregular bowel movements or an unbalanced diet can cause constipation which can be very irritating and painful. The reason for being constipated can really be anything: from different medical conditions, problems with your digestive system, various medicines, to an unhealthy diet. However, the number one reason why people suffer from this condition is because of what they eat.

There are many things you can do to prevent and eliminate constipation. This book offers plenty of balanced recipes to help ease constipation. This collection of delicious recipes is based on foods packed with fiber and other healthy nutrients. The recipes are very easy to prepare and you will see results in no time!

This book offers some great ideas to make your dining table simply irresistible. By adding enough fiber and some specific ingredients to your diet, you can reduce, and even heal constipation in a couple of days. Sound unbelievable? Well, I challenge you to try some of these recipes for a couple of days, and see for yourself!

This book includes many "constipation superfoods", and not only that, it has the power to improve your overall health.

46 MEAL RECIPES TO SOLVE YOUR CONSTIPATION PROBLEMS: IMPROVE YOUR DIGESTION THROUGH INTELLIGENT FOOD CHOICES AND WELL ORGANIZED MEAL RECIPES

1. Tender Venison Stew with Prunes

Ingredients:

21oz shoulder of venison, chopped into bite-sized pieces

1 cup of sour cream

2 ½ cup of beef broth

½ tsp of freshly ground black pepper

1 tsp of salt

5 tbsp of vegetable oil

4 large onions, finely chopped

7oz prunes, sliced

2 tbsp of fresh blackberries

1 cup of red wine vinegar

½ cup of whipping cream

1 bay leaf

Preparation:

In a small bowl, combine vinegar with bay leaf and blackberries. Pour the mixture over prunes and set aside for 30 minutes.

Heat up the oil over medium-high heat. Add chopped venison and briefly cook, 5-6 minutes. Now add chopped onions and continue to cook until translucent. Season with salt and pepper and gradually add beef broth, ½ cup at a time, stirring constantly.

When the meat is half tender, add prunes and vinegar mixture. Reduce the heat to a minimum and continue to cook for 45 minutes.

Stir in whipping cream and sour cream and serve warm.

Nutritional information per serving: Kcal: 380 , Protein: 49g, Carbs: 38g, Fats: 26g

2. Rice Omelet with Spring Onions

Ingredients:

4 tbsp of olive oil

3 whole eggs

1 cup of rice

4 large spring onions, chopped

½ tsp of freshly ground black pepper

1 tsp of salt

Preparation:

First you have to cook the rice. Use a package directions or simply combine one cup of rice with three cups of water. Bring it to a boil and give it a good stir. Reduce the heat to minimum and cook until the water evaporates. Remove from the heat and chill. Transfer to a serving platter.

Heat up the olive oil in a large saucepan, over a medium-high heat. Whisk the eggs in a bowl and season with some salt (about ¼ tsp). Pour the eggs in a skillet and fry for 2 minutes. Flip over and cook for one more minute. Remove from the heat and slice the egss into ½ inch thick strips.

Transfer to a bowl with rice. Add some more salt and pepper and give it a good stir.

Top with chopped onions and serve.

Nutritional information per serving: Kcal: 245 , Protein: 18g, Carbs: 40g, Fats: 22g

3. Vegetable Patties

Ingredients:

7oz carrot, sliced

3.4oz cauliflower, chopped

7oz broccoli, chopped

7oz kale, chopped

1 egg

3.5oz breadcrumbs

½ cup of all-purpose flour

2 tbsp of extra virgin olive oil

1 tsp of salt

For the sauce:

½ cup of liquid yogurt

½ cup of fat-free mayonnaise

¼ cup of sugar-free tomato sauce

Preparation:

Place the chopped vegetable in a deep pot. Add enough water to cover and one teaspoon of salt. Cook until fork tender. Remove from the heat and drain. Chill for a while and transfer to a food processor. Pulse to combine and place in a bowl.

Whisk in one egg and flour. Using your hands, shape one inch thick patties. Dip each pattie in breadcrumbs.

Heat up the olive oil in a large saucepan. Fry each patty for 3-4 minutes on each side and transfer to a serving platter.

Prepare the sauce by combine yogurt with mayonnaise and tomato sauce. Chill for a while and serve.

Nutritional information per serving: Kcal: 276 , Protein: 39g, Carbs: 41g, Fats: 30g

4. Broccoli Orecchiette

Ingredients:

1 pack (10oz) orecchiette

1lb broccoli

3.5 turkey breast fillet, thinly sliced

1 large onion, peeled and finely chopped

7oz button mushrooms, sliced

2 garlic cloves, crushed

½ cup of cooking cream

3 tbsp of extra virgin olive oil

1 tsp of salt

½ tsp of pepper

2 tbsp of grated parmesan

Preparation:

Heat up the olive oil in a large saucepan. Add chopped onion and stir-fry until translucent. Now add turkey breasts and continue to cook for 3-4 more minutes, stirring constantly. Now add garlic and button mushrooms, and stir well. Cook until the liquid evaporates and add cooking cream, salt, pepper, and chopped broccoli. If the mixture is too thick, you can add ¼ cup of vegetable stock. Reduce the heat, cover, and simmer for five more minutes.

Use a package instructions to prepare orecchiette. Drain and combine with broccoli sauce. Serve warm.

Nutritional information per serving: Kcal: 518 , Protein: 48g, Carbs: 53g, Fats: 24g

5. Stewed Turkey Breast with Celery Risotto

Ingredients:

1lb turkey breast meat, chopped into bite-sized pieces

7oz long grain rice

1 medium-sized onion, peeled and finely chopped

2 tbsp of melted butter

1.5oz celery root, sliced

1 tsp of nutmeg, ground

¼ cup of apple juice

A handful of fresh parsley

1 tsp of sea salt

½ tsp of freshly ground black pepper

Preparation:

Combine oil with butter in a large skillet. Heat up over medium-high heat and add onion and celery root. Stir-fry briefly, for 3-4 minutes and add turkey breast and continue to simmer adding about ¼ cup of water at a time. Now add apple juice, fresh parsley, and ground nutmeg. Give it a good stir and briefly boil. Remove from the heat.

Meanwhile, cook the rice. You can use a package direction to prepare your rice or simply place the rice in a deep pot and add four cups of water. Cook over medium heat until water has evaporated. Stir occasionally.

Combine rice with turkey breast sauce and serve warm. You can decorate with some more fresh parsley, but this optional.

Nutritional information per serving: Kcal: 413, Protein: 31g, Carbs: 39g, Fats: 20g

6. Steamed Chineese Spinach with Ginger

Ingredients:

14oz spinach

1 tbsp of sesame seeds

1 tsp of ginger, grated

2 tbsp of freshly squeezed lime juice

¼ cup of water

2 tbsp of olive oil

1 tsp of sesame oil

½ tsp of salt

Preparation:

Wash and clean spinach leaves. Roughly chop them and set aside.

Heat up olive oil and sesame oil in a large wok pan. Add chopped spinach and cover. Cook for ten minutes, uncover and add ginger, lime juice, sesame seeds, and water. Continue to cook for five more minutes.

Remove from the heat and serve.

Nutritional information per serving: Kcal: 209 , Protein: 5g, Carbs: 19g, Fats: 14g

7. Turkey Breast with Garlic and Broccoli

Introduction:

1lb turkey breast, sliced into one inch thick slices

1 tbsp of cayenne pepper

5 tbsp of vegetable oil

2 large carrots, sliced

1lb broccoli, sliced

2 garlic cloves, crushed

4 tbsp of extra virgin olive oil

Preparation:

Combine five tablespoons of vegetable oil with one tablespoon of cayenne pepper. Using a kitchen brush, spread the mixture over turkey breast. Set aside in the refrigerator for 30 minutes.

Meanwhile, place sliced carrot in a pot of boiling water. Add one teaspoon of salt and cook for ten minutes. Now add broccoli and continue to cook until fork tender. Remove from the heat and drain.

Heat up the olive oil in a large saucepan and add garlic, carrot and broccoli. Gently simmer for 5-6 minutes and add turkey breast. Cover and cook for 20 minutes.

Remove from the heat and serve.

Nutritional information per serving: Kcal: 175 , Protein: 29g, Carbs: 8.6g, Fats: 22g

8. Kidney Bean Salad with Eggs

Ingredients:

1 whole egg, boiled

1 cup of lettuce, finely chopped

½ cup of green beans, cooked

½ cup kidney beans, cooked

4 cherry tomatoes, halved

1 tsp of ground chili pepper

Few black olives, sliced

3 tbsp of extra virgin olive oil

½ tsp of salt

1 tbsp of fresh lemon juice

Preparation:

First you want to boil the egg. Gently place the egg into a pot with just enough water to cover. Bring to a boil and cook for 10 minutes. You can use a kitchen timer. After 10 minutes, drain the water and place the egg under the cold water. Peel and slice

Meanwhile, combine other ingredients in a large bowl. Add the olive oil, fresh lemon juice, and salt. Toss well to combine. Top with sliced eggs and serve.

To prevent the ingredients from changing the color in leftover salad, cover tightly with a plastic wrap. Keep in the refrigerator.

Nutrition information per serving: Kcal: 191 Protein: 45g, Carbs: 50g, Fats: 19.8g

9. Green Bean and Radish Salad with Olive Oil

Ingredients:

1lb green beans

7oz radish, sliced

5oz cherry tomatoes, halved

1 tsp of salt

Dressing:

4 tbsp of extra virgin olive oil

1 tsp of fresh mint, finely chopped

2 spring onions, chopped

2 tsp of freshly squeezed lime juice

½ tsp of salt

Preparation:

Wash and clean the beans and place in a deep pot. Pour enough water to cover and add one teaspoon of salt. Cook for 15-20 minutes. Remove from the heat and drain. Cool for a while and transfer to a serving bowl. Add halved tomatoes and sliced radish. Toss to combine.

In another bowl, combine all dressing ingredients. Drizzle over salad and serve cold.

Nutritional information per serving: Kcal: 200 , Protein: 1.1g, Carbs: 36g, Fats: 27g

10. Asian Curry Chicken with Prunes

Ingredients:

1lb chicken fillet, boneless and skinless

2 large red bell peppers

1 small green bell pepper

1 cup of freshly squeezed orange juice

4 prunes, pitted

1 cup of chicken broth

1 tbsp of ground curry

1 tsp of salt

¼ tsp of freshly ground black pepper

4 tbsp of vegetable oil

Preparation:

Season the meat with some salt and pour over the orange juice. Add prunes and marinate for 30 minutes. Remove the meat from the marinade and slice into bite-sized pieces.

Heat up the oil in a large wok pan and add chicken breast. Stir-fry for 3-4 minutes and add chopped, bell peppers, curry, pepper, and continue to cook for 2 more minutes.

Now add the chicken broth and bring it to a boil. Reduce the heat and simmer for 30 minutes.

Serve warm.

Nutritional information per serving: Kcal: 496 , Protein: 38g, Carbs: 40.5g, Fats: 26g

11. Arugula Salad with Parmesan

Ingredients:

10oz fresh arugula, torn

3.5oz grated parmesan cheese

Dressing:

¼ cup of extra virgin olive oil

2 tbsp of apple cider vinegar

1 tbsp of freshly squeezed orange juice

1 tsp of dijon mustard

1 tbsp of sour cream

Preparation:

Whisk together all dressing ingredients until fully combined. Chill for 30 minutes in the refrigerator.

Place arugula in a serving bowl. Add parmesan cheese and toss to combine.

Drizzle with dressing and serve cold.

This salad tastes even better when refrigerated overnight, but that is optional.

Nutritional information per serving: Kcal: 176 , Protein: 18g, Carbs: 21g, Fats: 19g

12. Fresh Vegetable Wraps with Greek Yogurt

Ingredients:

1 pound of chicken breast, boneless and skinless

2 cups of chicken broth

1 cup of fat-free Greek yogurt

1 cup of fresh parsley, chopped

½ tsp of sea salt

¼ tsp of ground pepper

4 cups of chopped lettuce

1 cup of diced tomato

½ cup of onion, sliced

1 package of whole grain tortillas

Preparation:

Combine chicken broth and chicken meat in a sauce pan over medium heat. Cover the sauce pan and allow it to boil. Cook for another 10-15 over medium-low heat. Remove from heat and drain. Let it stand for a while.

Chop the meat into bite size pieces. Meanwhile, in a large bowl, combine Greek yogurt, chicken meat, parsley, salt and pepper. Mix gently until the chicken is well coated.

Spread this mixture over tortillas and top with lettuce, tomato and onion. Roll and serve.

Nutrition information per serving: Kcal: 167, Protein: 21.5g, Carbs: 14.5g, Fats: 5g

13. Lentil Burgers with Garlic

Ingredients:

2 cups of lentils, pre-cooked

3 cloves of garlic, minced

½ cup of breadcrumbs

¼ cup of reduced fat parmesan cheese (freshly grated is best, but whatever you got will work)

1 egg, beaten

2 cups of water

½ cup of rice flour

salt and pepper to taste

Preparation:

1In a medium size bowl, mash lentils with folk then mix with garlic, breadcrumbs and cheese. Form into patties; set aside. Whisk egg and water in bowl; flour and salt & pepper in another bowl.

Coat each patty gently with flour mixture, dip into egg, then coat again with flour. Over medium-high heat in a large skillet, heat oil. Fry the burgers until lightly brown, about 2-3 minutes each side.

Serve on warm bread or in a pita with cilantro, yogurt, onion, tomatoes and whatever else you like – but this is optional!

Nutrition information per serving: Kcal: 195, Protein: 19.8g, Carbs: 16.1g, Fats: 6.7g

14. Creamy Winter Chicken

Ingredients:

1 pound of boneless chicken, chopped

1 2/3 cups of chicken broth

2/4 cup of chopped onions

½ cup of brown rice

½ cup of low-fat cottage cheese

3 tbsp of fat-free Greek yogurt

¼ tsp of salt

½ tsp of basil

¼ tsp of oregano

¼ tsp of thyme, crushed

1/8 tsp of garlic powder

1/8 tsp of pepper

Preparation:

Combine the chicken and onions into a skillet and cook between medium to high heat until chicken is cooked. This should take about 20-30 minutes.

Place chicken and onions into a large bowl and then add chicken broth, uncooked brown rice, basil, salt, oregano, thyme, garlic powder, pepper and cottage cheese. Mix up until everything is thoroughly combined.

3Place the mixture into an ungreased 1½ quart casserole dish with a tight fitting lid.

Preheat oven to 350 degrees. Bake covered for about 30 minutes, or until rice is done, stirring it several times during cooking.

Uncover the casserole dish and top with Greek yogurt.

Bake uncovered for about five more minutes until yogurt is completely melted. Garnish with parsley before serving.

Nutrition information per serving: Kcal: 198, Protein: 23.5g, Carbs: 16g, Fats: 5g

15. Sweet Potato and Mushroom Sliders

Ingredients:

1 large sweet potato

1 cup of fresh button mushrooms

1 cup of low-fat cottage cheese

3 egg whites

¾ cup of chia seeds

¾ of a cup of long grain rice

¾ of a cup of bread crumbs

1 tsp of tarragon

1 tsp of parsley

1 tsp of garlic powder

1 cup of chopped spinach

Preparation:

Pour 1 cup of water in a small saucepan. Bring it to boil and cook rice until it's slightly sticky. This should take about 10 minutes.

At the same time, cook chia seeds until soft in a separate pot. Finely chop mushrooms. Thoroughly rinse spinach.

Mix all the ingredients together in a large bowl. Put the bowl into the fridge to chill for 15 to 30 minutes. Take mixture out of the fridge and form into patties.

Make sure cooking surfaces are cleaned and greased before adding patties to prevent them from sticking. Fry each piece on a medium temperature for about 5 minutes on both side.

Nutrition information per serving: Kcal: 186, Protein: 22g, Carbs: 19g, Fats: 5.8g

16. Sweet Pumpkin Salad With Almonds

Ingredients:

1 cup of chopped pumpkin

1 cup of arugula

3 tbsp of chopped almonds

1 tsp of dry rosemary

½ tsp of dry thyme

Olive oil

Preparation:

Preheat the oven to 350 degrees. Grease the baking sheet with some olive oil. Spread the pumpkin and sprinkle with rosemary and thyme.

Bake for about 30 minutes.

Remove from the oven and allow it to cool for a while.

Meanwhile combine other ingredients in a bowl, add pumpkin, and some more olive oil. Serve.

Nutrition information per serving: Kcal: 180, Protein: 4g, Carbs: 28g, Fats: 2.1g

17. Hazelnut Quinoa with Cranberries

Ingredients:

1 cup of quinoa, cooked

3 tbsp of hazelnuts, roasted

½ cup of fresh parsley

1 small onion, peeled and chopped

2 garlic cloves

¼ tsp of salt

5 tbsp of olive oil

1 cup of button mushrooms, sliced

¼ cup of cranberries, dry

Preparation:

Combine the hazelnuts, parsley, salt and 3 tbsp of olive oil in a food processor.

Blend well for 30 seconds.

Heat up the remaining olive oil in a large skillet. Add chopped onion and garlic. Stir well and fry for several minutes, until nice light brown color.

Add cooked quinoa, button mushrooms, and mix well. Cook for 5 more minutes, until the water evaporates. Remove from the heat and transfer to a bowl. Add hazelnut mixture and ¼ cup of cranberries.

Mix well and serve warm.

Nutrition information per serving: Kcal: 160, Protein: 17g, Carbs: 31g, Fats: 12g

18. Lentil Stew with Turmeric

Ingredients:

10oz lentils

tbsp of canola oil

1 medium-sized carrot, peeled and sliced

1 small potato, peeled and chopped

1 bay leaf

¼ cup of parsley, finely chopped

½ tbsp of turmeric powder

Salt to taste

Preparation:

Melt the butter in a medium-sized skillet. Add sliced carrot, chopped potato and parsley. Mix well and stir-fry for about five minutes.

Now add the lentils, 1 bay leaf, some salt and chili powder. Add about 4 cups of water and bring it to a boil. Reduce the heat, cover and cook until the lentils soften.

Sprinkle with some parsley before serving.

Nutrition information per serving: Kcal: 313, Protein: 36g, Carbs: 42g, Fats: 28g

19. Breakfast Creamy Mozzarella Tricolore

Ingredients:

2 large tomatoes, sliced

3.5oz mozzarella, sliced

1 medium-sized avocado, halved and stone removed

3 tbsp of extra virgin olive oil

½ tsp of salt

1 tsp of apple cider vinegar

½ tsp of dried thyme, crushed

½ tsp of stevia

Preparation:

Wash and slice tomatoes. Place them on a serving platter.

Cut avocado in half and remove the stone. Slice thinly and make a layer over tomatoes. Top with mozzarella.

In a small bowl, whisk together olive oil, apple cider, thyme, salt, and stevia. Drizzle over tricolore and serve.

Nutrition information per serving: Kcal: 340 Protein: 16.5g, Carbs: 5.8g, Fats: 31g

20. Warm Strawberry Coconut Flakes

Ingredients:

¼ cup of flaked coconut, lightly toasted

1 cup of almond milk (you can use coconut almond milk for some extra flavor)

1 tbsp of chia seeds

1 tbsp of almonds, minced

1 tbsp of coconut oil

1 tsp of strawberry extract, sugar-free

½ tsp of stevia

Preparation:

Preheat the oven to 350 degrees. Line some baking paper over a baking sheet and grease with melted coconut oil.

Pour the flakes onto the sheet and toast for 10-15 minutes. Remove from the oven and transfer to a bowl.

Add almond milk, minced almonds, chia seeds, strawberry extract, and stevia. Give it a good stir and serve warm.

Nutritional information per serving: Kcal: 175 , Protein: 3.1g, Carbs: 8.6g, Fats: 19g

21. Baked Zucchini with Blue Cheese Drizzle

Ingredients:

1 medium-sized zucchini, sliced lengthwise

2 large eggs

¼ cup of almond milk

½ cup of almond flour

2 garlic cloves, crushed

1 tsp of dried oregano, crushed

½ cup of gorgonzola

1 tsp of salt

½ tsp of pepper

¼ cup of extra virgin olive oil

Preparation:

Preheat the oven to 350 degrees. Grease a quarter-sized sheet pan with some olive oil and set aside.

Combine the remaining oil with crushed garlic, oregano, and pepper. Set aside.

Slice the zucchini lengthwise and sprinkle with some salt. Set aside for 5-7 minutes. Rinse well and pat dry. Arrange a single layer in a baking dish. Using a kitchen brush, spread the olive oil mixture over each zucchini slice and bake for 20 minutes.

Meanwhile, whisk together eggs, almond milk, and almond flour. Beat well with an electric mixer on high until well incorporated. Spread this mixture over zucchini and continue to cook for five more minutes.

Place gorgonzola in a microwave for two minutes. Drizzle over zucchini and serve warm.

Nutritional information per serving: Kcal: 340, Protein: 19g, Carbs: 7.3g, Fats: 35g

22. Garlic Shiitake Casserole

Ingredients:

1lb shiitake mushrooms, whole

6 eggs

2 medium onions, peeled

3 garlic cloves, crushed

¼ cup of olive oil

½ tsp of sea salt

¼ tsp of freshly ground black pepper

Preparation:

Preheat the oven to 350 degrees. Spread 2 tbsp of olive oil over an eighth-sized baking sheet. Place the shiitake on a baking sheet. Bake for about 10-12 minutes. Remove from the oven and allow it to cool for a while. Lover the oven heat to 200 degrees.

Meanwhile, peel and finely chop the onions. Separate egg whites from yolks. Slice shiitake into ½ inch thick slices and place in a bowl. Add chopped onions, olive oil, egg whites, crushed garlic, salt and pepper. Mix well.

Spread this mixture over a baking sheet and bake for another 15-20 minutes.

Nutritional information per serving: Kcal: 319, Protein: 41g, Carbs: 14g, Fats: 34g

23. Sweet Asparagus with Parmesan Cheese

Ingredients:

1lb fresh asparagus, woody ends trimmed

2 medium onions, peeled and finely chopped

2 small jalapeno peppers, sliced

1 cup of vegetable stock

¼ cup of fresh lime juice

1 tsp of pure orange extract, sugar-free

5 tbsp of extra virgin olive oil

1 tsp of dried rosemary, crushed

Preparation:

Heat up the olive oil in a large saucepan. Add chopped onions and stir-fry for 2-3 minutes, or until translucent.

Place jalapeno peppers, lime juice, orange extract, and rosemary in a food processor. Add about ½ cup of vegetable stock and pulse until smooth. Pour the mixture into a frying pan and reduce the heat to minimum. Simmer for ten minutes.

When most of the liquid has evaporated, add trimmed asparagus and the remaining vegetable stock. Bring it to a boil and simmer until asparagus are fork tender.

Serve warm.

Nutritional information per serving: Kcal: 180, Protein: 4.9g, Carbs: 7g, Fats: 41g

24. Stripped Vegetables in Wok

Ingredients:

1 pound of button mushrooms, sliced

1 medium red bell pepper, cut into strips

1 medum green bell pepper, cut into strips

7-8 cauliflower florets

½ cup of parmesan cheese

7-8 brussel sprouts, halved

1 tbsp fresh tomato sauce, sugar-free

1 fire-roasted tomato, roughly chopped

1 tsp of salt

4 tbsp of extra virgin olive oil

Preparation:

Thoroughly wash and slice mushrooms lengthwise.

In a large wok pan, heat up the olive oil over a medium-high temperature. Add cauliflower florets and brussel sprouts and cook for ten minutes, stirring constantly. Now add stripped peppers, fire-roasted tomato, salt, tomato sauce, and parmesan cheese. Give it a good stir and cook for ten more minutes.

Now you can add mushrooms and continue to cook for 5-7 more minutes. Give it a final stir and serve warm.

Nutritional information per serving: Kcal: 313, Protein: 18.9g, Carbs: 14g, Fats: 32g

25. Hot Chili Cauliflower Stew

Ingredients:

2 pounds of cauliflower florets

1 tbsp chili pepper, ground

1 tablespoon of vegetable oil

6 oz tomato paste, sugar-free

2 jalapeno peppers, cut into strips

1 large tomato, roughly chopped

1 large onion, peeled and finely chopped

1 cup of fresh button mushrooms, sliced

¼ tbsp of salt

1 bay leaf

2 ½ cups vegetable broth

1 tsp of dry thyme

3 garlic cloves, crushed

Preparation:

Take a frying pan and set it over high heat. Heat up the vegetable oil and add the cauliflower florets to it. Cook, stirring constantly, until properly brown. Transfer to a deep pot. In the same pan, fry the onions, turning the heat to medium. Cook the onions for 5 minutes.

Now add jalapeno peppers, tomato paste, chili pepper, garlic and salt. Continue to cook for 3-4 minutes. Transfer to a pot.

Add the remaining ingredients and cover with a lid. Set the heat to minimum and cook for one hour.

Nutritional information per serving: Kcal: 180, Protein: 13g, Carbs: 25g, Fats: 8.9g

26. Crustless Creamy Spinach Pie

Ingredients:

1 pack (9 ounces) of fresh spinach, chopped

4 whole eggs

½ cup of coconut milk

2 oz of crumbled Feta cheese

¼ cup grated Parmesan cheese

½ cup shredded Mozzarella cheese

3 tbsp of vegetable oil

1 tsp of salt

½ tsp of black pepper

Preparation:

Preheat the oven to 350°F. Lightly grease a baking dish with vegetable oil and set aside.

Whisk the eggs thoroughly in a mixing bowl. Gradually whisk in the milk and beat well on high. Add parmesan and continue to beat until well combined. Set aside.

Place the chopped spinach in the greased baking dish and add crumbled Feta cheese. Pour in the egg mixture and cover the other ingredients completely.

Bake for about 40 to 45 minutes or until the cheese has melted and lightly browned.

Remove from the oven and chill for 10-15 minutes before serving.

Nutritional information per serving: Kcal: 190, Protein: 15g, Carbs: 8g, Fats: 20g

27. Lamb's Lettuce with Fresh Goat's Cheese and Tomatoes

Ingredients:

5 cherry tomatoes, whole

A handful of black olives

1 medium-sized onion, peeled and sliced

3.5 oz fresh goat's cheese

2 radishes, sliced

3.5 oz of lamb's lettuce

2 tbsp of freshly squeezed lime juice

3 tbsp of extra virgin olive oil

Salt to taste

Preparation:

Place the vegetables in a large bowl. Add olive oil, goat's cheese, fresh lime juice and some salt to taste. Toss to combine.

Nutritional information per serving: Kcal: 225, Protein: 18.5g, Carbs: 10g, Fats: 35g

28. Cheesy Button Mushrooms

Ingredients:

2 small zucchinis, sliced lengthwise

½ cup of cottage cheese

1 cup of lamb's lettuce

1 cup of cherry tomatoes

½ cup of button mushrooms, sliced

1 tsp of salt

½ tsp of freshly ground black pepper

2 tbsp of olive oil

Preparation:

Wash and pat dry the zucchini with some kitchen paper. Slice lengthwise.

Use a large grill pan and grease it with some olive oil. Heat up over medium-high heat and sliced zucchinis. Grill for 3-4 minutes on each side, remove from the heat and chill for a while.

Meanwhile add mushrooms into the grill pan and grill until the liquid evaporates. Remove from the heat and chill for a while.

Place lamb's lettuce, cottage cheese, and cherry tomatoes in a large bowl. Add grilled zucchini, mushrooms, and season with salt and pepper. Toss to combine and serve.

Nutritional information per serving: Kcal: 220, Protein: 27g, Carbs: 14g, Fats: 24g

29. Vegge Cabbage Rolls

Ingredients:

1 pound of fresh cabbage leaves

3 large eggs

½ cup of cauliflower, pre-cooked and finely chopped

1 medium-sized tomato

1 tbsp of fresh parsley, chopped

¼ tsp of sea salt

¼ tsp of black pepper, ground

5 tbsp of olive oil

Preparation:

Gently place the eggs in a deep pot. Add enough water to cover and bring it to a boil. Cook for 10 minutes. Remove from the heat, cool for a while and peel. Place in a medium-sized bowl and mash with a fork. Set aside.

Wash, peel and finely chop the tomato. Place it in a large bowl. Combine the eggs, chopped cauliflower, parsley, salt, and pepper. Add about two tablespoons of olive oil to this mixture. Place about two tablespoons of this mixture in the center of each cabbage leaf. Roll up nicely tuck in the ends.

Now add the remaining oil in a deep pot. Carefully place the rolls in a pot and add about 1 cup of water. Cover and cook over a medium-high heat for about 20 minutes.

Nutritional information per serving: Kcal: 240, Protein: 29g, Carbs: 27g, Fats: 42g

30. Warm Broccoli Slaw

Ingredients:

12 oz bag broccoli slaw

½ cup of brussel sprouts, halved

½ cup of cauliflower, chopped

A hanful of finely chopped kale

3 tbsp of sesame oil

1 tsp of ginger, grated

½ tsp of salt

¼ cup of goat milk yogurt

Preparation:

Heat up the oil in a large skillet. Add brussel sprouts and chopped cauliflower. Cook for 10-15 minutes, stirring constantly.

Stir in brocoli slaw, grated ginger, salt, and kale. Add about ¼ cup of water and continue to cook for another 10 minutes. When the water has evaporated, stir in yogurt and remove from the heat.

Serve warm.

Nutritional information per serving: Kcal: 214, Protein: 9g, Carbs: 13g, Fats: 15g

31. Vegetarian Kebab

Ingredients:

1 lb rib cauliflower florets, halved

2 large onions, grated

5 tbsp of extra virgin olive oil

½ tsp of red pepper, crushed

½ tsp of dried oregano

¼ tsp of salt

¼ tsp of ground black pepper

1 tbsp of tomato sauce

2 cups of lukewarm water

1 large tomato, sliced into wedges

½ green pepper, chopped

1 cup of plain yogurt, or sour cream

Preparation:

First, put the onions into a blender and blend until smooth. Transfer the liquid from the blender into a large bowl, and remove the remaining pulp.

Cut the cauliflower florets and slice it into bite-sized pieces.

Combine the spices with two tablespoons of olive oil and onions. Stir well. Now add the cauliflower and stir all together. Cover the lid and set aside.

Now, preheat the remaining olive oil over a medium temperature. Add the tomato sauce and stir well. If you're a fan of spicy food, you can add a pinch of crushed chili pepper. This, however, is optional. Now add the water, a pinch of salt, and gently simmer for a couple of minutes. Remove from the heat and set aside.

Meanwhile, heat up 2 tablespoons of vegetable oil and add the cauliflower. Stir-fry for about ten minutes. Now add the tomato sauce and onions. Stir well and cook for another five minutes. Set aside.

Place the cauliflower pieces onto a serving platter, top with tomato and pepper, and serve with some yogurt or sour cream.

Enjoy!

Nutritional information per serving: Kcal: 190, Protein: 12g, Carbs: 21g, Fats: 22g

32. Cold Gazpacho

Ingredients:

1 pound of fresh tomatoes, peeled and finely chopped

3 large cucumbers, finely chopped

3 spring onions, finely chopped

1 medium-sized red onion, finely chopped

1 tbsp of tomato paste, sugar-free

½ tsp of salt

1 tbsp of ground cumin

¼ tsp of pepper

Fresh parsley, for serving

Preparation:

Preheat the non-stick frying pan over a medium-high temperature. Add the onions and stir-fry for 3-4 minutes. Now add the tomatoes, tomato paste, cucumber, cumin, salt, and pepper. Cook for another five minutes, or until caramelized.

Add three cups of lukewarm water, reduce the heat to minimum and cook for about 15 minutes. Now add about

1 cup of water and bring it to a boil. Remove from the heat and serve with fresh parsley.

Serve cold.

Nutritional information per serving: Kcal: 320, Protein: 12.5g, Carbs: 70g, Fats: 13g

33. Sweet Almond Patties

Ingredients:

1lb cauliflower florets, sliced

7oz almonds, toasted

1 cup of almond milk

1 egg

1 tsp of sea salt

1 tbsp of almond butter

1 cup of almond flour

½ cup of parsley, finely chopped

½ cup of plain yougurt

Vegetable oil

Preparation:

Place cauliflower florets in a deep pot. Add enough water to cover and bring it to a boil. Cook until fork tender. Remove from the heat and transfer to a bowl. Add one teaspoon of salt, almond milk, and almond butter. Mash until a smooth puree. Set aside.

Finely chop the almonds and combine with cauliflower puree. Add almond flour, eggs, and parsley. Mix until well combined. Using your hands, shape 1-inch thick patties.

Preheat some oil over a medium-high heat. Fry each patty for about 2-3 minutes on each side.

Nutritional information per serving: Kcal: 322, Protein: 17g, Carbs: 18g, Fats: 28g

34. Creamy Cheese Lettuce Wraps

Ingredients:

3 large iceberg lettuce leaves

1 medium-sized tomato

½ red bell pepper, finely chopped

1 garlic clove, crushed

1 tsp of dry oregano

2 tbsp of grated goat's cheese (can be replaced with some other cheese)

1 tsp of extra virgin olive oil

½ tsp of salt

2 tbsp of finely chopped parsley

Preparation:

Combine together tomato, chopped pepper, crushed garlic clove, oregano, olive oil, salt, and parsley in a large bowl. Spread some of the mixture over each lettuce leaf and wrap. Secure with a toothpick and serve.

Enjoy!

Nutritional information per serving: Kcal: 133, Protein: 7g, Carbs: 11g, Fats: 21g

35. Braised Greens with Fresh Mint

Ingredients:

3.5oz fresh chicory, torn

3.5oz wild asparagus, finely chopped

3.5oz Swiss chard, torn

A handful of fresh mint, chopped

A handful of rocket salad, torn

3 garlic cloves, crushed

¼ tsp of freshly ground black pepper

1 tsp of salt

¼ cup of fresh lemon juice

Olive oil

Preparation:

Fill a large pot with salted water and add greens. Bring it to a boil and cook for 2-3 minutes. Remove from the heat and drain.

In a medium-sized skillet, heat up 3 tablespoons of olive oil. Add crushed garlic and stir-fry for about 2-3 minutes.

Now add the greens, salt, pepper, and about half of the lemon juice. Stir-fry the greens for five more minutes.

Remove from the heat. Season with more lemon juice and serve.

Nutritional information per serving: Kcal: 55, Protein: 4g, Carbs: 7g, Fats: 8g

36. Warm Caponata

Ingredients:

7oz brussel sprouts, chopped into bite sized pieces

1 zucchini, sliced

1 medium-sized onion, peeled and chopped

2 large, fresh tomatoes, roughly chopped

3.5 oz cabbage, shredded

1 medium-sized chili pepper

2 stalks of celery

3 tbsp of olive oil

1 tbsp of red wine vinegar

Salt to taste

1 tsp of stevia

½ tbsp of basil, dry

Preparation:

Chop zucchini into bite-sized pieces and season with some salt. Allow it to stand for about 5 minutes and rinse well.

Meanwhile, heat up the olive oil over a medium heat. Add the onions and stir-fry for 2-3 minutes. Now add celery, basil, stevia, salt, vinegar, and tomatoes. Continue to cook for 2 more minutes.

Transfer to a deep pot and add other ingredients. Add about one cup of water and cook for about 20 minutes over high temperature.

Nutritional information per serving: Kcal: 160, Protein: 11g, Carbs: 28g, Fats: 9g

37. Creamy Manicotti

Ingredients:

5 crepes

¼ cup of coconut oil

3oz coconut flour

2pts coconut milk

8.8oz ricotta cheese

3oz grated Parmesan cheese

5oz fresh spinach, torn

Seasoning to taste

Preparation:

Preheat the oven to 350 degrees.

Bring the coconut oil, flour and milk slowly to a boil, whisking constantly until thickened. Put half of the sauce into a bowl and mix with ricotta, parmesan, spinach, and seasoning to taste.

Lay a crepe on the work surface. Spoon out about 1/5 of the mixture and place it on crepe. Roll up the crepe and place it on a baking sheet. Repeat the process until you have used all the ingredients.

Bake for 10 minutes, remove from the oven and serve.

Nutritional information per serving: Kcal: 500, Protein: 31g, Carbs: 11.5g, Fats: 50g

38. Sweet tomato soup

Ingredients:

2oz tomato, peeled and roughly chopped

Ground black pepper to taste

1 tbsp of celery, finely chopped

1 onion, diced

1 tbsp of fresh basil, finely chopped

Fresh water

Preparation:

Preheat the non-stick frying pan over a medium-high temperature. Add the onions, celery, and fresh basil. Sprinkle some pepper and stir-fry for about 10 minutes, until caramelized.

Add the tomato and about ¼ cup of water. Reduce the heat to minimum and cook for about 15 minutes, until softened. Now add about 1 cup of water and bring it to a boil. Remove from the heat and serve with fresh parsley.

Nutrition information per serving: Kcal: 25 Protein: 0.7g, Carbs: 4.9g, Fats: 0.9g

39. Chocolate Protein Bars

Ingredients:

1 cup of toasted almonds, finely chopped

½ cup of cocoa butter

½ cup of sweetener, powdered

2 tablespoons of chia seeds

¼ cup of raw cocoa powder

3 egg whites

¼ cup of coconut milk

Preparation:

Combine the ingredients in a bowl and mix well to combine. Shape the balls using your hands and refrigerate for about 30 minutes.

Nutritional information per serving: Kcal: 260, Protein: 11g, Carbs: 9g, Fats: 28g

40. Chef salad to go

Ingredients:

3 large eggs

½ cucumber, sliced

1 small tomato, roughly chopped

1 cup of fresh lettuce, torn

1 small green pepper, sliced

½ tsp salt

1 tbsp of lime juice

3 tbsp of olive oil

Preparation:

Hard boil the eggs for 10 minutes. Remove from the heat, rinse and chill for a while. Gently peel and slice each egg. Transfer to a large jar.

Now, combine the vegetables in a glass jar. Add the meat and mix well. Season with salt and some lime juice. Seal the lid and you're ready to go.

Nutritional information per serving: Kcal: 55, Protein: 7g, Carbs: 2.8g, Fats: 11.3g

41. Super Healthy Beet Greens Salad

Ingredients:

8 oz leek, chopped into bite-size pieces

Handful of beet greens

1 large tomato, chopped

2 garlic cloves, finely chopped

3 tbsp of vegetable oil

A few mint leaves

½ tsp of salt

½ tsp of red pepper

½ tsp of Cayenne pepper

Preparation:

Heat up some vegetable oil in a large skillet. Stir-fry the garlic for 2-3 minutes, or until lightly charred. Now add leek, salt, pepper, and cayenne pepper. Cook for ten minutes, over medium heat, stirring constantly. Remove from the heat and transfer to a bowl.

Add a handful of beet greens, chopped tomato, and fresh mint. Toss well to combine and serve.

Nutritional information per serving: Kcal: 133, Protein: 2.1g, Carbs: 15g, Fats: 15.5g

42. Ginger Peach Smoothie

Ingredients:

1 cup of coconut milk

1 tbsp of coconut oil

1 tbsp of chia seeds

1 tsp of ginger, ground

2 tsp of sweetener, powdered

1 tsp of pure peach extract, sugar-free

Preparation:

Combine the ingredients in a blender and pulse to combine. You can add some ice cubes, but this is optional. Serve cold.

Nutritional information per serving: Kcal: 417, Protein: 6g, Carbs: 10g, Fats: 41g

43. Cherry Avocado Smoothie

Ingredients:

½ ripe avocado, chopped

1 cup of coconut water, sugar-free

1 tbsp of fresh lime juice

1 tsp of sweetener, powdered

1 tsp of pure cherry extract, sugar-free

Preparation:

Place the ingredients in a food processor and pulse to combine. Serve cold.

Nutritional information per serving: Kcal: 210, Protein: 4.5g, Carbs: 18g, Fats: 16g

44. Fresh Avocado Smoothie

Ingredients:

½ avocado, roughly chopped

1 cup of coconut milk

1 tbsp of walnuts, chopped

1 tsp of vanilla extract, sugar-free

1 tsp sweetener, powdered

A handful of ice cubes

Preparation:

Place the ingredients in a blender and pulse to combine. Serve cold.

Nutritional information per serving: Kcal: 212, Protein: 8g, Carbs: 12g, Fats: 36g

45. Coconut Yogurt with Chia Seeds and Almonds

Ingredients:

1 cup of coconut yogurt

3 tbsp of chia seeds

1 tsp of toasted almonds, finely chopped

2 tsp of sweetener, powdered

Preparation:

For this easy recipe, combine 3 tbsp of chia seeds with 1 cup of coconut yogurt, 1 tsp of ground almonds and 1 tbsp of honey. Use a fork or an electric mixer to get a smooth mixture. Allow it to cool in the refrigerator.

You can combine ¾ cup of coconut yogurt with ¼ cup of rice yogurt for extra flavor.

Nutritional information per serving: Kcal: 312, Protein: 14g, Carbs: 44g, Fats: 41g

46. Coco Pudding

Ingredients:

2 cups of unsweetened coconut milk (you can use almond milk for extra flavor)

¼ cup of toasted coconut flakes

1 tbsp walnuts, finely chopped

1 tbps of hazelnuts, finely chopped

1 tsp of stevia, powdered

1 tsp of cinnamon, ground

½ tbsp of sugar-free vanilla extract

Preparation:

In a medium sized saucepan bring 2 cups of coconut milk to boil. Gently stir in the coconut flakes and reduce the heat to minimum. Cook until they double in size and then add walnuts, hazelnuts, stevia, cinnamon, and vanilla extract.

Give it a good stir and cook for five more minutes.

Remove from the heat and chill for a while. Transfer to serving bowls and cool in the refrigerator for about 30 minutes before serving.

Nutritional information per serving: Kcal: 193, Protein: 3.8g, Carbs: 6g, Fats: 12g

ADDITIONAL TITLES FROM THIS AUTHOR

70 Effective Meal Recipes to Prevent and Solve Being Overweight: Burn Fat Fast by Using Proper Dieting and Smart Nutrition

By

Joe Correa CSN

48 Acne Solving Meal Recipes: The Fast and Natural Path to Fixing Your Acne Problems in Less Than 10 Days!

By

Joe Correa CSN

41 Alzheimer's Preventing Meal Recipes: Reduce or Eliminate Your Alzheimer's Condition in 30 Days or Less!

By

Joe Correa CSN

70 Effective Breast Cancer Meal Recipes: Prevent and Fight Breast Cancer with Smart Nutrition and Powerful Foods

By

Joe Correa CSN

www.ingramcontent.com/pod-product-compliance
Lightning Source LLC
Chambersburg PA
CBHW062149020426
42334CB00020B/2552